I0421205

true

Contents

Type 2 Diabetes Treatment

How to Treat Type 2 Diabetes Fast — The Proven Type 2 Diabetes Treatment

Quick Start Guide

"The Tried-And-True Eating System That Helps You Achieve Normal, Healthy Blood Sugar, Body Weight and Energy"

Sunny Lam MES, BSCH

Copyright 2015

LIMIT OF LIABILITY AND DISCLAIMER:

This manual is based on personal experience and is designed to provide information about the subject matter covered. Every effort has been made to make it as complete and accurate as possible. However, there may be mistakes both typographical and in content. Website URL's and content can change overnight

— so if you click through to a site and it's not there, please contact the author so that it can be corrected.

The author shall have neither liability nor responsibility to any person or entity with respect to any loss or damage caused or alleged to be caused directly or indirectly by the information covered in this manual.

This book is not meant to be used, nor should it be used, to diagnose or treat any medical condition. For diagnosis or treatment of any medical problem, consult your own physician. The publisher and author are not responsible for any specific health or allergy needs that may require medical supervision and are not liable for any damages or negative consequences from any treatment, action, application or preparation, to any person reading or following the information in this book.

References are provided for informational purposes only and do not constitute endorsement of any websites or other sources.

TRADEMARKS:

Any trademarks, service marks, product names or named features are assumed to be the property of their respective owners, and are used for reference only.

SHARING THIS DOCUMENT:

I ask that you please respect the work I do by not giving away or reselling this guide. I sincerely thank you for that respect!

Chapter 1 - Can You Free Yourself? And the Answer Is Yes

If you're serious about leading a normal, pain-free, happy life...

Without type 2 diabetes...

Without the constant frustration of trying to keep your blood sugar under control...

Without losing your eyes, fingers and toes to blood sugar rot and nerve damage...

Without constant prickling pain keeping you up at night...

Without having to exercise two hours a day or like some kind of Olympic athlete...

Without packing on the pounds from insulin shots...

Or turning into a sloth from the constant energy slumps and fatigue....

If you want to enjoy life and food again...

And if you have the desire to regain control of your life...

Then you can DO this...

Listen, you have to do this if you want to make your life better than before because it is possible...

If you want to do all the things you love like hiking, jogging, sports, hanging out with friends, gardening or spending time with the family or your bouncing grand-kids...

I know it's possible because I did it and many others have used similar principles to do so as well...

Chapter 2 - Why Act Now? Here's Why...

The World Health Organization pegs type 2 diabetes as becoming the 7th leading killer by 2030...

And it's the side effects which are the main reason diabetics end up in the morgue or in an early grave...

Such as...

- Heart disease: **death rates are at least 1.7 times higher for type 2**

diabetics [1] than non-diabetics...

- Amputation: **60% of lower limb amputations happened to diabetics** [2]...

- Permanent Blindness or Eye Problems: **nearly 28.5%+ of diabetics had damaged vision** in 2008[3]...

- Kidney Disease: **type 2 diabetes was the cause of kidney failure in 44% of cases** in 2011 and 228,924 people were hooked to a dialysis machine like it was a "ball and chain"[4]...

- Poor Memory and Foggy Brain: A study of 141 women aged 63[5] showed that **constant high blood sugar has a "negative" impact on your memory and learning**...

- And more...

The prescription drugs in use often hurt us in the long run with their side effects... causing everything from nausea or upset stomach to intestinal bleeding...

---

[1] ADA, "Statistics About Diabetes: American Diabetes Association," American Diabetes Association, February 19, 2015. Accessed Monday, February 23, 2015, http://www.diabetes.org/diabetes-basics/statistics/.

[2] ADA 2015

[3] ADA 2015

[4] ADA 2015

[5] Kerti, Lucia, et al. "Higher glucose levels associated with lower memory and reduced hippocampal microstructure." Neurology 81.20 (2013): 1746-1752.

Often they don't even get your blood sugar to a level you need in a reliable way...

Worst of all?...

A 14 year study of 3336 patients[6] found that **diabetics treated with insulin had a 329% increase in death rates from any cause**...

Which is worse than being untreated (222%) or using drugs (128%)...

There has to be a better way...

And there is...

IF you follow a tried-and-true eating System that will help you get a grip over your blood sugar situation...

You'll no longer be a slave to your blood sugar and all the frustrations that come with it...

No more sleepless nights...

You'll look and feel better and more energized than you have in years...

And you'll be smarter and wiser for solving your blood sugar challenges by yourself...

---

[6]Berard, Emilie, et al. "14-Year Risk of All-Cause Mortality According to Hypo-glycaemic Drug Exposure in a General Population." PloS one 9.4 (2014): e95671. http://www.ncbi.nlm.nih.gov/pmc/articles/PMC3994099/.

Able to enjoy all the things you couldn't while you were trapped by type 2 diabetes...

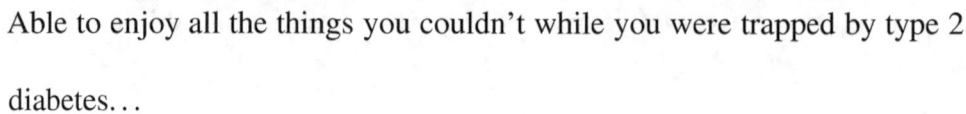

Chapter 3 - Why Has Type 2 Diabetes Been Such a Mystery Until Now?

It took me over 7 years to figure out the real dirt behind type 2 diabetes... and that's what led to the core System that you have in your hands today...

After pouring through hundreds of scientific articles, books and reports, I've assembled the latest information to help you heal your body and bring your blood sugar back under control...

It's the same information which I used to heal myself...

And you'll learn the core steps of that System in the following pages...

Now I want you to know that neither you or I are to blame for what happened to us...

There's so much rotten or confusing information out there that most people can't figure out what to believe...

People don't know the truth about how to manage their blood sugar, counter type 2 diabetes deadly side effects, avoid weight gain and constant fatigue...

There are two myths that may be ruining your life, your blood sugar, your weight and your energy...

The first is that lowering blood sugar is the only goal...

The second is that you should get 45-65% of your calories or energy from carbs...

None of these are true and you'll learn why soon enough...

Chapter 4 - Life After Type 2 Diabetes Is Like...

Imagine achieving normal blood sugar and insulin levels, while while gaining crystal clear mental focus, nearly limitless energy and amazing confidence and a positive mood...

All those aches and pains in your joints fade away...

Your allergies practically vanish...

And you never have to touch a single unit of insulin or take any blood sugar drugs with dangerous side effects ever again...

You forever stop worrying that you'll have to amputate your hands, feet, fingers or toes and become a cripple...

Your appetite becomes half of what it was before...

And even "temptation" doesn't even bother you any more...

Your stomach will feel incredible and things like acid reflux become a thing of the past...

Plus your weight will reach amazing healthy levels that you're happy enough to show off to your friends and family...

Chapter 5 - Here's The Big Picture...

First you'll learn what you need for the success and freedom you'll achieve by managing your type 2 diabetes and blood sugar today...

Then you'll learn the core "Insulin Freedom" System which is a simple, step-by-step process you'll follow to achieve the insulin and blood sugar levels you desire...

Each step will be explained in as much crystal clear detail as a quick start guide can give you and... in a way that doesn't overwhelm you either...

You'll learn more about the advanced techniques, beginner tips every diabetic should know and the major mistakes to avoid when you explore the "full" System later on...

Chapter 6 - Here's What You Need to Manage Your Type 2 Diabetes...

There's six areas of preparation that we'll quickly run through to get you ready for this new life without complications, frustrating blood sugar highs and lows, weight gain and constant tiredness...

The first is your mind, the second is your body, the third is gear, the fourth is time, the fifth is money and the sixth is your emotions...

Let's start with the mental prep...

Mental Preparation...

Now look, you must want to save yourself otherwise why are you reading this right?

Can you afford to wait until you start going blind, or the nerve damage and pain becomes so great that they have to lop off your toes or fingers?...

And I doubt you want to be chained to a dialysis machine for the rest of your life...

If you need a reality check, you can re-read the previous intro chapters or Google some horror stories...

It's not pretty...

Listen, when you solve your type 2 diabetes yourself you're more likely to stick with this for the long haul and the more information you have, the higher the chances of your success — it's a scientifically proven fact that well informed and motivated people can double their chances of managing their type 2 diabetes[7]...

So here's what you're going to do...

Write your goals down right now...

Write out all the good and bad of what you're doing...

Write down your commitment to treating your type 2 diabetes over the next 4,

---

[7]Osborn, Chandra Y., and Leonard E. Egede. "Validation of an Information Motivation Behavioral Skills model of diabetes self-care (IMB-DSC)." Patient education and counseling 79.1 (2010): 49-54.

Rachmani, Rita, et al. "Treatment of high-risk patients with diabetes: motivation and teaching intervention: a randomized, prospective 8-year follow-up study." Journal of the American Society of Nephrology 16.3 suppl 1 (2005): S22-S26.

12 or 16 weeks...

Write up a plan of what you'll be doing each week... a schedule of when you'll shop for food, cook, exercise and save for leftovers...

And most importantly...

Keep these goals and plans handy in a notebook — paper or digital or stuck on the fridge...

Use a calendar to mark your shopping trips...

Buy canned and storable foods for flexibility or "rush" days...

The key is to make it as easy as possible to help yourself... the clearer things are, the less road blocks and excuses there are not to save yourself and your health...

Track your progress every week, updating your journal or notebook at least twice a week...

Record your victories over type 2 diabetes, the "wins", the "happy" things...

Track your exercises...

All of this tracking will make it easier when you do cut or drop your meds and insulin at the right rate and time...

Plus it keeps you motivated...

Know that I'm in your corner and that you can contact me for help...

Physical preparations are next...

Physical Preparation

You don't have to do any kind of serious labour to get started with this system... short of cleaning out cupboards and trashing junk food...

Using this System means you don't have to exercise hard or long or at all if you really don't want to... though it helps...

You'll learn more about the benefits of exercise on your type 2 diabetes when you explore the full System later on...

Next comes the gear or materials...

Material Preparation

Here are the "things" you need to get or use... like making your kitchen healthy...

This is THE major step... The line in the sand you must cross...

You want to drop the "toxic" foods you've been eating up 'till now from your fridge, cupboards or hidden stashes...

Toss it out...

Toss out the soy oil, corn oil and high heated oils if possible because that'll make your type 2 diabetes (and heart) worse off and switch to butter, lard or coconut oil...

You'll learn more about why later on...

If you live with others who don't follow this lifestyle, create a separate storage area for your food...

Then stock up on the healthy food...

What else?...

Buy a notebook to track your progress remember?...

Or use a digital system like Evernote...

Grab an app or web app to track your carbs, protein and fat...

My recommendations?

MyFitnessPal first, Fitday and SELF Nutrition Data...

All three work, though MyFitnessPal has the largest food database and SELF provides the most nutrition information...

Plus grab a pedometer if that helps...

If you have one, you can count your steps... the average person should take

7,000 to 10,000 steps a day for good health... this'll help count those stairs you take...

Otherwise you'd count time... 10,000 steps takes around 30 to 40 minutes...

And finally you may want to buy two or three sets of workout clothes so you have no excuse not to exercise...

Next is time prep...

Time Preparation

Now not everyone needs time management tools — that'll depend on you...

If you like constant reminders because your type 2 diabetes is giving you brain fog, then you can set these up on your phone or computer or mark them in your day book...

Include reminders about not overeating, what foods to avoid and what supplements or meds you have to take...

Include a few reminders about exercising if you're inclined to... at most 3 to 4 times a week... and it doesn't have to be longer than 30 minutes or an hour...

Track your blood sugar numbers and/or weight on a calendar...

Mark the day you started this System... and the day you hit your "dream" or "ideal" blood sugar numbers...

You'll be filled with glee as you watch your numbers come down over time...

Next is the dollar investment you need to make in yourself...

How much money are you going to spend on healing yourself of type 2 diabetes forever?

How much is that worth to you?

Most diabetics spend on average $13,700 per year on medical costs on top of their food costs...

That's $1,141 a month in medical bills and supplies... so tack on your cost of food at that point and do the math...

Eating well doesn't have to cost you more than $3,600 to $6,000 a year if you spend say $300, $400 or $500 a month on food and certain vitamins or supplements, which you learn about in the full System...

You don't have to spend on organic, natural or local food — even the regular supermarket versions of the food you'll learn about are fine...

You also have the added bonus of getting rid of nearly any or all of your medical bills too...

Eating well is an investment in your health that pays off for your body and your wallet...

If you're not willing to invest in saving yourself you can just stop reading right now and keep on doing what you've been doing...

Seriously, this is a no-brainer...

Finally you need to psych yourself up emotionally...

Emotional Preparation

Your friends and family might wonder why you've changed your eating habits and lifestyle...

They might keep tempting you with dire sweets and "bad, white" carbs during the holidays...

Best way to deal with this is to tell them straight up what you're trying to get your blood sugar and type 2 diabetes under control...

Explain to them why it's important to you and what the deadly results are if you don't...

And get them to help you stick to it...

You can also make your commitment and progress public on your own social media profiles if you use any... that'll also help you stick to your goals because you don't want to be seen as a flake...

It's also a common issue for a lot of discouraging responses from people around you, even your family doctor...

Don't let those people or words get to you... harden yourself and prove them wrong...

This is your life and your health... living and eating the way everyone else did got you into this mess (through no fault of your own) and you're going to get yourself out...

And you will!

If you feel alone or isolated then you can find others like yourself who have gone through the same thing...

Find the support groups... or gain access to the How To Treat Type 2 Diabetes Fast community by investing in the full System...

There will be many others who have gone through what you have including myself...

Share your story, gain inspiration, acquire help when you need it plus access all the free resources available only to those who are part of the HTDF community...

Coming Up...

Now, in the next chapter you'll finally learn about the core System that uses the Insulin Freedom Principle...

Chapter 7 - Here's the Plan to Master Your Blood Sugar...

The "Insulin Freedom" Plan is the core of the System and lifestyle and it can be customized to suit your unique needs especially if you use the advanced techniques and beginners tips from the "full" System which you can discover later on...

The core System takes things both "slow and fast" because your diet is for the long term and we're getting you to learn new "habits" while setting aggressive goals you can meet every week...

You want to make sure you have your doctor or health team backing you up just in case...

Now the System is based on the "Insulin Freedom Principle" which goes something like this (part of it anyway)...

80% of the fat that clogs your arteries, liver and pancreas comes mostly from carbs NOT the fat you eat[8]...

It's this clogging that actually wrecks your blood sugar "control" and leads to type 2 diabetes...

Think about it... why do people who drink soft drinks gain weight when there's not an ounce of fat in the drinks themselves?

Ever wonder?

What you just learned helps explain why that happens...

By following the System you're going to "unclog" your insulin controls and signals so you never have to worry about see-sawing glucose, blindness, amputation, dialysis machines, weight gain or energy slumps ever again...

This is the key part of the improved version of the System I used to master my own blood sugar within a year without starving myself and without much heart pumping exercise (no, really)...

It's many who've used similar principles and I know it'll work for you...

Plus calorie counting is totally not required...

---

[8]Paoli, A., et al. "Beyond weight loss: a review of the therapeutic uses of very-low-carbohydrate (ketogenic) diets." European journal of clinical nutrition 67.8 (2013): 789-796.

Less work for you!

So let's move onto...

Week 1

Summary of This Week's Steps

- You're going to cut down the amount of total carbs you eat to 150 g...

- Switch the kind of carbs you eat to the "good" carbs not "bad, white" carbs...

- You're going to increase the amount of fat you eat to 60-100 g...

- Start cutting down your meds and insulin...

- Avoid dairy and cheese for now...

Chop Your Total Carbs to 150 g...

Why chop it to 150 grams?...

Because this starts you down the road through the "Fat Burning" Zone...

It hops right back to the "Insulin Freedom Principle" because 80% of the carbs you eat produces almost all of that insulin wrecking fat[9] (which also damages your heart, promoting cancer and a lot of other diseases[10])...

Now, 150 g is about 3 fist-sizes of carbs where every fist is about 40-50 g... or the size of a baseball...

Works pretty well for estimating protein too...

Then...

Switch From "Bad, White" Carbs to "Good" Carbs...

Now the Insulin Freedom Principle is a good start however there are "good" carb foods that you can eat which are mostly fibre and another special kind of

[9]Paoli et al. 2013

[10]Joseph Mercola, "A High-Carb Diet May Increase Your Risk of Dementia," Mercola.com, March 13, 2014. Accessed Monday, March 16, 2015, http://articles.mercola.com/sites/articles/archive/2014/03/13/high-carb-diet.aspx.

Romieu, Isabelle, et al. "Carbohydrates and the risk of breast cancer among Mexican women." Cancer Epidemiology Biomarkers & Prevention 13.8 (2004): 1283-1289.

Perlmutter, David. "Rethinking Dietary Approaches for Brain Health." Alternative and Complementary Therapies 20.2 (2014): 73-75.

Roberts, Rosebud O., et al. "Relative intake of macronutrients impacts risk of mild cognitive impairment or dementia." Journal of Alzheimer's Disease 32.2 (2012): 329-339.

Ronnemaa, E., et al. "Impaired insulin secretion increases the risk of Alzheimer disease." Neurology 71.14 (2008): 1065-1071.

Crane, Paul K., et al. "Glucose levels and risk of dementia." New England Journal of Medicine 369.6 (2013): 540-548.

Agrawal, Rahul, and Fernando Gomez Pinilla. " 'Metabolic syndrome' in the brain: deficiency in omega3 fatty acid exacerbates dysfunctions in insulin receptor signalling and cognition." The Journal of physiology 590.10 (2012): 2485-2499.

Grabenhenrich, Linus B., et al. "Higher glucose levels associated with lower memory and reduced hippocampal microstructure." Neurology 83.1 (2014): 102-102.

carb that you'll learn about in the full System...

You don't want to eat high starch vegetables or grains...

That means NO white/brown/red rice, no potatoes of any kind, no white/whole/enriched wheat and no other grains if at all possible...

You definitely shouldn't be eating any of these by Week 3 or 4...

I'd drop the steel cut oatmeal too... that's "white" and too easy to digest...

What you want to eat are beans, vegetables, nuts and seeds if at all possible...

With seeds and nuts you can have as much as 6 ounces or 170 g a day to start with...

Plus drop the squashes, yams and similar high starch vegetables too... until you've got your blood sugar in check in Weeks 4 to 6...

Use non-starchy cooked veggies or tofu for hearty stews like...

- Eggplant

- Tomatoes

- Onions

- Garlic

- Mushrooms

- Peppers

- Beans

- Zucchini

Green veggies have special "phyto-sterols" and chemicals that repair and "shield" your body from disease and fix your type 2 diabetes...

They've been shown to lower type 2 diabetes risk by 14%[11] for example when compared to meat and potatoes...

Also NO sweetened drinks or fruit juice of any kind should be used either... that includes those meal replacement shakes which are practically pure sugar with some added vitamins...

... It's like drinking heroin or cocaine when it comes to a diabetic...

And you should eat less dried fruit because 1/2 a cup is as sweet as eating a whole cup of regular fruit...

... I'd avoid fruit in general except berries...

If you're eating beans, nuts and seeds, the dietary fibre doesn't have to be counted toward the 150 g limit for the week (or later weeks) unless your blood

---

[11]Carter, Patrice, et al. "Fruit and vegetable intake and incidence of type 2 diabetes mellitus: systematic review and meta-analysis." Bmj 341 (2010).

sugar keeps spiking to dangerous levels and refuses to go down... in those cases, count the fibre as well...

More troubleshooting tips can be found in the full System...

Next is...

Eat More Healthy Fat!...

You now know that "bad, white" carbs is the main reason for your type 2 diabetes... however fat is what will also help you control your food cravings by making you feel full faster and for much, much longer...

This is also one of the keys to my success and the success of many others who've following this kind of System...

Anyway, fat gives you double the amount of energy that protein or carbs would give you and... eating more fat helps to switch you into a "fat burner" mode...

You want get around 60-100 g of fat in your diet... roughly 50% of your energy calories in a day...

Now if you're eating nuts and seeds like I suggested you'll gain roughly 82 g of fat from 6 ounces or 170 g of nuts...

Plus all the amazing micronutrients and minerals that most people lack in their diets these days...

Your other options include...

- Avocado

- Cheese (if you don't want to listen to the next step)

- Coconut, coconut flakes and/or coconut milk

- Olive oil (only if you can find fresh, reliable brands)

- Ghee

- Butter

Also remember to...

Start Cutting Down the Meds and Insulin...

This is an area where you must consult a doctor...

The drops in blood sugar you'll experience if you use this System and any of the advanced techniques means that your blood sugar might plummet too fast and far causing anything from faintness or dizziness to shock IF you're using your meds at regular doses...

You'll also require less and less insulin as the days and weeks go by...

So redo the math with your doctor's help...

It's time to start figuring this all out this week or earlier...

Furthermore...

Avoid the Milk, Dairy and Cheese...

If you can avoid all milk, dairy and cheese... especially milk and dairy... then do it... because no matter how small an amount you eat, the blood sugar spikes are giant...

If you like living dangerously you could add them back after Week 4 when you've mastered your blood sugar...

If you're in it for the long haul you're better off leaving these out forever...

Next up is...

_____

Week 2

Summary of This Week's Steps

- Set Your Carb Limit to 51 to 100 g Per Day...

- Increase The Amount of Fat Eaten By Another 50 g (Optional)...

Eat Only 51 to 100 g Carbs Per Day...

Now you're building on your efforts from last week... by lowering your carbs per day to 2 fist-sizes or fistfuls per day or 51 to 100 g...

This is taking you further into the "Fat Burning" Zone, which causes your body to burn more and more of its stored fat and "unclogging" the insulin-blood-sugar control systems...

If you've been eating enough fat (and maybe protein) you'll find this very easy to do no matter what kind of diabetic you are or for however long you've been one...

Increase The Amount of Fat Eaten By Another 50 g (Optional)...

Now if for some reason you're having trouble or feeling hungry still, increase the amount of nuts and seeds you eat by up to 3 ounces (putting you to a maximum of 9 ounces per day or 255 g)...

Or if you're not following the advice of eating nuts and seeds then you could add more fats like butter or coconut oil... another 50 to 54 g... about a quarter cup...

If you're a highly active athlete or body builder you might want to add the above and another 50 g of fat anyway (or 1-2 ounces of nuts)...

Week 3 and Week 4

Summary Of These Week's Steps

- Set Your Carb Limit to 30 to 50 g Per Day...

- Increase The Amount of Fat Eaten By Another 50 g (Optional)...

Set Your Carb Limit to 30 to 50 g Per Day...

Or one fist-size or fistful roughly...

Now you're really strolling through the final stages of the "Fat Burning" Zone...

Just so you know, you won't be here forever unless you want to be...

More will be explained in the full System if you want to know why...

At this stage you'll be transforming into a "Fat Burner" and there'll be a wildfire inside of your body as the fat that's been "clogging" your organs and sabotaging your insulin system is boiled away...

This is only possible as long as you're eating enough fat to feel full and avoiding the "bad, white, heroin" like carbs you learned about in Week 1...

Increase The Amount of Fat Eaten By Another 50 g (Optional)...

Again if you're still feeling hungry then it means you're not eating enough fat...

So up the amount of nuts by another 1-3 ounces until you feel full or...

Increase the amount of fat by another quarter cup or 50 to 55 g... whether that's butter or coconut oil...

Though I highly recommend you use nuts and seeds...

For the average person, 60 to 80 grams of fat a day is usually enough...

If you're an athlete, body builder or highly active person or labourer you can add the above plus another 1-3 ounces of nuts, or 50-55 g of fat (or quarter cup)...

Finally...

By the end of Week 4, most diabetics of less than 5 years should have hit their "sweet spot" for insulin and blood sugar...

Most of the diabetic side effects should be gone or on their way out the door...

Your weight should be at the ideal level for you...

And you should feel energized, alive and vibrant...

For diabetics of 5, 13, 20 or 40+ years, your blood sugar numbers, energy and mood will be improving during this period though you may not see any outward signs of weight change...

Don't worry... the fat's still being burned away inside of your body... the process hasn't reached your hips or belly yet that's all...

Week 5 and Beyond

Summary Of These Week's Steps

- Increase Your Carb Limit to 51 - 100 g Per Day Starting Week 5 (Optional)...

- Increase Your Carb Limit to 101 - 150 g Per Day Starting Week 12 (Optional)...

You'll continue with what you were doing in Weeks 3 and 4...

By Week 6, most diabetics of 5+ years have often hit the minimum time "milestone" to see their ideal blood sugar results...

Again the longer you've been diabetic, the more fat build up you need to burn through...

So be patient...

If you've had type 2 diabetes for 13, 20 or 40+ years it may take you as long as 4 to 6 months to finally reach your ideal blood sugar levels...

Again it varies with the person and their situation... Some may take as long as 9 months to a year...

Compared to being a diabetic for years or decades however this is actually a very short amount of time...

IF you're using the advanced techniques to speed up your blood sugar and type 2 diabetes control (found in the full System), even a long term diabetic will typically hit their best blood sugar level by the 6 month mark... (these advanced techniques can speed up your progress by 50% or more...)

Increase Your Carb Limit to 51 - 100 g Per Day Starting Week 5 (Optional)...

If you're satisfied that your insulin, blood sugar, weight and energy are completely under control then you can experiment with increasing your "good" carb limit to 51 to 100 g per day...

You'll want to keep avoiding the refined, "bad, white" carbs of course that we talked about in Week 1...

Instead you'll add more vegetables, beans, nuts and seeds into your diet...

Increase Your Carb Limit to 101 - 150 g Per Day Starting Week 12 (Optional)...

If your type 2 diabetes and blood sugar are doing really well even after increasing your "good" carbs to 51-100 g per day then you can experiment with increasing it to 101 to 150 g per day now...

Same advice of course as above...

NOTE: Even with dietary fibre included I never eat above 130 grams of carbs per day... excluding the dietary fibre means I typically never eat above 100... as a kind of guideline...

Conclusion

If you've reached Week 12 and you're seeing the blood sugar, weight and energy control that you've been yearning for...

You've now mastered the core System and a new lifestyle that will give you the health you deserve...

Compared to everyone else you're a lean, mean sugar and fat burning machine who is in better health than 99% of the people out there...

Congratulations!

You're set for life!

No one can take away this knowledge and these habits!

_____

If you want to get in touch with me, you can reach me in the following ways...

Email: health.fenix@gmail.com

Web Site: http://healthfenix.com

_____

For Those Keen Souls Who Want Even **Faster**, More Potent **Results** In the Shortest Amount of Time...

You'll want the complete System including...

- the 7 Most Effective Ways To Achieve Normal Healthy Blood Sugar, Weight and Energy Levels At Your Finger Tips (two of them are shockingly simple 2059-year old ways for managing your type 2 diabetes that the medical establishment doesn't bother to tell you about...)

- The 11 beginner tips that every diabetic should know...

- Access to 71 of the most commonly asked questions covering everything from results and risks... to drugs, blood sugar, blood pressure, cholesterol and weight... Allowing you to solve your most thorniest problems with a flip of a page...

- The 5 most common mistakes many diabetics make when trying to manage their type 2 diabetes...

- The Type 2 Diabetes Supplement Survival Guide (covering over 30 vitamins, minerals and supplements that could help you manage your blood sugar quicker and more easily...)

- The Treat Type 2 Diabetes — Quick and Easy Meals cookbook... (with over 99 mouth watering, diabetic friendly recipes...)

- And more...

You'll want to check out the full version at http://how-to-treat-diabetes.com/...

www.ingramcontent.com/pod-product-compliance
Lightning Source LLC
Chambersburg PA
CBHW061932280526
45787CB00004B/1572